TABLE OF CONTENTS

INTRODUCTION

Have you reached the point where you are giving up on your ill child out of discouragement? Even worse, you might consider yourself a failure. Well, it makes sense that despondency would set in during this difficult time. It matters how you choose to handle this!

Taking care of a sick child is challenging and demanding a lot of the time. How much can you discuss with your doctor to completely understand the illness your sick child is experiencing in order to give them the care they need? The appropriate action you take will enable you to manage and cope with your child's illness more effectively.

You can better control the situation by expressing any worries you may have and by asking questions about how your child is being cared for.

It is essential and advantageous to learn more about the condition, particularly its preventative and control strategies, in order to manage your child's illness.Rest confident that this publication has useful advice that would REALLY benefit you. You'll be glad you did.

In order to effectively care for your sick child, you must communicate with your doctor and have a thorough understanding of the illness your child is dealing with. You'll be better equipped to manage and cope with your child's condition as a result.

Inform the doctor about your child's symptoms and medical background in a transparent and open manner.

Ask inquiries and voice any worries you may have regarding how your child is being treated.

Follow your doctor's advice for treatment, including any medication and therapy provided.

Observe your child's development, taking note of any changes in symptoms or adverse effects from the medication.

To make sure that all of your child's requirements are being met, coordinate with other healthcare team members including nurses and specialists.

Be proactive in looking for extra help or options for you and your kid, such support groups or home health care.

Organize and keep current all of your child's papers and medical records.

To track your child's growth, make sure to make routine checkups and follow-up appointments with the doctor.

Having knowledge about your child's illnesses

Research the specific condition or disease your child has been diagnosed with, including its causes, symptoms, and treatment options.

Ask your child's doctor to explain the diagnosis in detail, including any test results, and to answer any questions you may have.

Understand the potential long-term effects of the condition on your child's health and development.

Learn about any lifestyle changes or accommodations that may be necessary to help manage your child's condition, such as special diets or physical therapy.

Find out if there are any support groups or community resources available for families dealing with similar conditions, as these can provide valuable information and emotional support.

Keep yourself informed of the latest medical research and developments related to your child's condition, and discuss any new findings with your child's doctor.

Be aware of any warning signs or symptoms that may indicate a worsening of your child's condition, and know when to seek medical attention.

Keep track of your child's treatment plan and progress, including any medications, therapies, and special instructions from the doctor.

Factors that expose children to illnesses

There are several factors that can expose children to illnesses. Some of these include:

Close proximity to other children: Children in daycare, school, or other group settings are more likely to be exposed to illnesses because they come into contact with more people.

Poor hygiene: Children who don't practice good hand hygiene or who don't wash their hands regularly are more likely to get sick.

Lack of vaccines: Children who are not vaccinated are more susceptible to certain illnesses.

Exposure to environmental pollutants: Children living in areas with poor air or water quality may be more likely to get sick due to exposure to pollutants.

Exposure to secondhand smoke: Children exposed to secondhand smoke are at an increased risk of respiratory illnesses.

Poor nutrition: Children with poor nutrition are more susceptible to illnesses.

Lack of sleep: Children who don't get enough sleep are more likely to get sick.

Stress: Children who experience a lot of stress may be more susceptible to illnesses.

It's important to note that these are some of the most common

factors that can expose children to illnesses, but there are

many other factors that can also contribute. Consult a

pediatrician for more information on how to prevent illnesses

and keep your child healthy.

CHAPTER TWO: WHAT DISEASES AFFECT KIDS THE MOST?

Children's illnesses can be brought on by a number of things,

such as allergies, bacterial and viral infections, and

environmental factors. Children frequently contract the flu,

colds, strep throat, ear infections, and stomach viruses.

Children can also get unwell from having some chronic

disorders like asthma and eczema. Children's illnesses can also

be influenced by environmental factors including pollution

exposure and passive smoking. For more information or if you have concerns about something serious, speak with a pediatrician. This article would cover a few common illnesses. Take your time to absorb the knowledge presented here, which will motivate you to manage your sick child's condition more actively.

Common Cold

Does your child have watery eyes and a blocked or runny nose? Is he coughing and sneezing? He might be fighting a cold. Infants and young children frequently contract colds. The toddler may also have a fever if his body feels heated.

What to keep your child away from:

Keep your child away from crowded locations: A playground is one such spot. A Little Dirt Is Good for You, of Course. Both you and your children will benefit from playing outside. Sure, they could end up a little dirty, but all that exercise and perhaps even the dirt is doing wonders for their immune system. Encourage your children to play outside, get messy, and explore since doing so helps them develop stronger immune systems. While necessary, this should only be done to a limited extent.

All that outside exercise can also help to facilitate restful sleep. And that matters for a child's immune system. Lack of sleep reduces essential molecules that help fight illnesses in adults and kids. This suggests that your youngster may be more susceptible to developing a stuffy nose.

Avoiding ill people:

How can children avoid cold from ill people?

Children can avoid getting a cold from ill people by practicing good hygiene. This includes washing their hands frequently with soap and water, avoiding close contact with people who are sick, and avoiding touching their eyes, nose, and mouth. Additionally, it is also important for parents and caregivers to keep children away from crowded places during cold and flu season. Encourage children to cover their nose and mouth with a tissue or their elbow when they cough or sneeze, and to throw away used tissues immediately. If a child does become ill, they should stay home and avoid contact with others until they have fully recovered.

Other kids:

Children can be encouraged by their parents or other adults to cover their mouth and nose when they cough or sneeze, and to throw away used tissues right away. Children should also be educated not to share personal belongings with other children, such as towels, combs, and eating utensils, as this could be one of the quickest ways to spread the virus.

CHAPTER THREE : FIGHTING ROSEOLA

Roseola is a common viral infection that primarily affects young children, typically between the ages of 6 months and 2 years old. It is caused by the human herpesvirus 6 (HHV-6) or human herpesvirus 7 (HHV-7). Symptoms include a high fever that lasts for 3-5 days, followed by a rash that appears on the trunk of the body and spreads to the limbs. The rash is usually pink or red in color and can be itchy. Other symptoms may include swollen lymph nodes, runny nose, cough, and sore throat.

The infection is usually self-limiting and resolves on its own within a week. Treatment typically includes fever management, such as giving the child acetaminophen or ibuprofen. Most children recover without any complications.

History of roseola

The history of roseola, also known as sixth disease or exanthema subitum, is not well-documented. The condition was first described in the medical literature in the late 19th century, but it is likely that the infection has been present in humans for much longer. The viruses that cause roseola, human herpesvirus 6 (HHV-6) and human herpesvirus 7 (HHV-7), were not identified until the late 20th century.

The name "roseola" comes from the Latin word "roseus," which means "rose-colored," referring to the characteristic rash that appears on the trunk and limbs of infected children. The term "exanthema subitum" means "sudden rash" in Latin.

Roseola is most commonly seen in children under the age of 2, but can also occur in adults, especially in people with compromised immune systems. The infection is typically self-limiting and resolves on its own, but in rare cases, can lead to serious complications such as encephalitis or seizures.

Research on roseola has primarily focused on identifying the viruses that cause the infection and understanding how they spread, as well as developing diagnostic tests and vaccines.

Prevention and Treatment of roseola in children

Prevention of roseola in children is primarily through avoiding exposure to the virus. Since it is a common infection in young children, it is difficult to completely avoid exposure to the viruses that cause it. However, good hygiene practices such as frequent handwashing and avoiding close contact with infected individuals can help reduce the risk of infection.

There is currently no specific treatment for roseola. The infection is usually self-limiting and resolves on its own within a week. Treatment typically includes fever management, such as giving the child acetaminophen or ibuprofen to reduce fever and discomfort. Over-the-counter antihistamines can also be used to relieve itching.

In rare cases, roseola can lead to serious complications such as encephalitis or seizures. In these cases, treatment will focus on managing the symptoms and complications of the infection. For example, antiviral medications may be prescribed to help manage encephalitis, and anticonvulsants may be used to control seizures.

It's important to consult with a pediatrician if you suspect your child has roseola, especially if your child has a high fever, to rule out other serious illnesses.

It's also important to keep in mind that roseola is a contagious infection, so parents or caregivers of infected children should take precautions to prevent spreading the infection to others.

Although the exact cause of chickenpox is unknown, it is thought to have been a part of human populations for a very long time. Varicella-zoster virus (VZV), the virus that causes chickenpox, is closely linked to the herpes zoster virus, which causes shingles. Given that the virus is not known to naturally exist in any other animal, it is most likely that it has evolved particularly to infect humans.

Does your child have a fever and red, itchy rashes on their body and faces? Over a few days, the chickenpox rash grows and eventually develops into blisters. Scratched locations may create scars if they become infected. In healthy children, chickenpox is frequently a common and minor infection. Due of its high contagiousness, HPV can spread swiftly by direct touch or airborne droplets from an infected person.

What to Do: If your child has chickenpox, keep him home from daycare or school to prevent the disease from spreading to other children; trim his fingernails to stop him from scratching; consider letting him wear gloves at night; and give him a cool bath to relieve itching.

⬜ In addition, take your child to the doctor if they experience any of the following symptoms: tremors, loss of muscle coordination, a stiff neck, dizziness, confusion, vomiting, rapid heartbeat, shortness of breath.

⬜ Finally, take your child to the doctor if the rash spreads to the eye or becomes extremely red or tender.

How to prevent and treat measles in children.

Although its exact origin is unknown, it is thought to have been a part of human populations for a very long time. The measles virus (MV), a member of the paramyxovirus family, is what causes the disease. When an infected individual coughs or sneezes, the virus easily spreads through the air and is very contagious. Given that the virus is not known to naturally exist in any other animal, it is most likely that it has evolved particularly to infect humans.

Measles is a dangerous viral infection that is highly contagious, especially in young children. The measles, mumps, and rubella (MMR) vaccine is the most effective strategy to prevent measles in children. To stop the infection from spreading, a child who has measles should not be around other children. In the event that a child is found to have the measles, supportive care, such as rest, water, and fever-reducers, may be given. A youngster could occasionally require hospitalization due to problems like pneumonia or encephalitis. Immune globulin may be administered to a youngster who has been exposed to the measles but is not immune to stop the infection.

Strep throat is an infection caused by the bacterium Streptococcus pyogenes. It is most commonly seen in children between the ages of 5 and 15. Strep throat is spread through respiratory droplets that are produced when an infected person talks, coughs or sneezes. Children can also become infected by touching objects or surfaces that have been contaminated with the bacteria and then touching their mouth or nose. Other risk factors include exposure to large crowds, having a weakened immune system, and not practicing good hygiene.

Treatment of Strep throat in children

The treatment for strep throat in children typically includes antibiotics to clear the infection. Penicillin and amoxicillin are commonly prescribed antibiotics for strep throat in children. These medications are usually given for 10 days.

It is also important for children to get plenty of rest, drink fluids, and relieve pain and fever with over-the-counter medications such as ibuprofen or acetaminophen.

To help relieve sore throat and other symptoms, children can also use:

Saltwater gargle

Popsicles or ice chips

Humidifier to add moisture to the air

Soft or cold foods

It's also important for children with strep throat to stay home from school or daycare until they have been on antibiotics for at least 24 hours and are feeling better to prevent the spread of the infection to others.

It's always good to follow up with a pediatrician if the child is not improving or if the symptoms worsen.

Ear infections in children are caused by a buildup of fluid in the middle ear, which can become infected by bacteria or viruses. The most common cause of ear infections in children is a blocked or swollen Eustachian tube, which connects the middle ear to the back of the throat. This can be caused by colds, allergies, or other upper respiratory infections.

Symptoms of ear infections in children include ear pain, difficulty sleeping, difficulty hearing, tugging or pulling at the ear, and crying more than usual. If a child has a fever or is in severe pain, it is important to seek medical attention.

Treatment for ear infections in children typically includes antibiotics if the infection is caused by bacteria, pain relievers, and decongestants to relieve symptoms. In some cases, a doctor may also recommend ear drops to help reduce inflammation and pain. In more severe cases, a tube may be placed in the eardrum to help drain the fluid and prevent future infections. In all cases, it's important to follow the doctor's instructions and complete the full course of treatment.

Prevention of ear infections include avoiding exposure to second hand smoke, keeping up with vaccinations, and keeping the child's nasal passages clear by using saline nasal sprays or drops.

Stomach viruses, also known as viral gastroenteritis, are caused by a variety of viruses such as norovirus, rotavirus, and adenovirus. These viruses can be spread through contaminated food or water, close contact with an infected person, or by touching contaminated surfaces and then touching your mouth. Symptoms include nausea, vomiting, diarrhea, and stomach cramps.

Treatment for a stomach virus typically includes rest and hydration to replace fluids lost due to vomiting and diarrhea. Over-the-counter medications such as bismuth subsalicylate

(Pepto-Bismol) can help with symptoms, but it's important not to take any medication that could worsen your diarrhea, such as non-steroidal anti-inflammatory drugs (NSAIDs) or antidiarrheal drugs.

It's important to practice good hygiene to prevent the spread of the virus, such as washing your hands frequently, especially after using the toilet, and avoiding close contact with people who are sick.

Most people recover from a stomach virus within a few days to a week, but in some cases, dehydration may require medical treatment. If you're experiencing severe symptoms, have difficulty keeping liquids down, or are unable to drink enough fluids to stay hydrated, it's important to seek medical attention.

A common respiratory virus called the respiratory syncytial virus (RSV) can make kids sick, especially those under the age of two. Since RSV has no specific medication, managing the virus mostly entails reducing symptoms.

The following actions can be taken to aid in managing RSV in kids:

Drink a lot of water to avoid being dehydrated.

Use over-the-counter drugs to reduce temperature and pain, such as acetaminophen or ibuprofen.

Utilize a cool mist humidifier to reduce coughing and congestion

As tolerated, encourage rest and activities

Keep the child away from other kids, especially sick ones.

Consult a doctor if the youngster is not improving after a few days or is experiencing trouble breathing.

It's also important to know that there is a preventative therapy for high-risk infants, such as premature infants, called palivizumab(Synagis), which is a monthly injection during the RSV season.

It's important to note that if your child is showing signs of severe illness such as difficulty breathing, chest retractions, or bluish skin color, you should seek medical attention immediately.

It's important to note that these are some of the most common illnesses that affect children and there are many other illnesses that can affect children as well. Consult a pediatrician if you suspect your child has an illness or if they are experiencing symptoms that are severe or persistent.

Chapter Hand, foot, and mouth disease (HFMD)

Hand, foot, and mouth disease (HFMD) is a common viral infection that primarily affects children. The symptoms include fever, sore throat, and a rash on the hands, feet, and inside the mouth. The infection is usually mild and self-limiting, but can be more severe in infants and young children. In most cases, bronchiolitis will resolve on its own within a few weeks. However, in severe cases, hospitalization may be necessary for further treatment. Over-the-counter medications such as cough and cold remedies should not be used in children with bronchiolitis as they have not been proven to be effective and may be harmful.

To manage HFMD in children, the following steps can be taken:

Provide adequate fluids to prevent dehydration.

Offer over-the-counter pain relievers such as ibuprofen or acetaminophen to relieve fever and pain.

Keep the child at home until the fever has subsided for at least 24 hours, to prevent the spread of the infection.

Use a soft toothbrush and avoid acidic or spicy foods to minimize mouth soreness.

Keep the child's fingernails short to reduce the risk of secondary skin infections from scratching.

Clean and disinfect frequently touched surfaces, such as toys, doorknobs, and bathrooms, to prevent the spread of the virus.

It's important to note that a visit to a doctor is generally not necessary, but if the child is not drinking enough fluids, has severe mouth sores, or has difficulty breathing, it's best to seek medical attention.

What You Should Do:

▢ Keep Your Child Hydrated with Fluids Like Water and Vitamin C-Rich Juices

▢ Stay away from Smoky Environments.

▢ If your child starts wheezing for the first time, or if his breathing becomes labored, or if he appears lethargic, lacks energy, or refuses to eat, take him to the doctor very once.

Are your child's hands, feet, or buttocks covered with rashes or blisters? Does your child have a fever, sore throat, or severe mouth ulcers? He might be infected with hand, foot, and mouth. This can occasionally turn into something more serious. Check your child's hands for blisters

What to Do: ⬚ If your child has HFMD, let the school, daycare center, or baby care facility know. Keep your youngster hydrated and at home to prevent the infection from spreading to other kids. Give him plenty of fluids and water; change to a soft diet (like porridge) as mouth ulcers can be excruciatingly painful; assist your child in getting plenty of bed rest; take precautions to stop the spread of HFMD at home, like cleaning all toys and other items that your child comes into contact with; and take your child to the doctor right away if you suspect he has the disease.

IDIOPATHIC SEIZURES

A youngster experiencing a febrile seizure may pass out, stiffen up, fall over unexpectedly, or have jerking arms and legs. A clinched jaw and rolling of the eyeballs back in the skull are further signs.

Idiopathic seizures in children are seizures that occur without an identifiable underlying cause. They are also known as primary or genetic seizures. These types of seizures are caused by abnormal electrical activity in the brain. Some possible causes of idiopathic seizures in children include genetic mutations, abnormal brain development, and unknown factors that affect the brain's electrical activity.

Treatment for idiopathic seizures in children typically involves the use of anti-seizure medication. The specific medication used will depend on the type of seizures the child is experiencing and their individual response to the medication. The goal of treatment is to control seizures and prevent them from recurring. In some cases, surgery may be recommended if medication is not effective.

It's also important to ensure that the child has a safe environment, with minimal risks of injury, and to maintain a seizure diary to understand the pattern and triggers of the seizures.

It's also important for the child and family to receive education and support about the seizures, and about how to handle seizures when they happen, such as how to safely help a child during a seizure and how to prevent injury. Regular follow-up with a pediatric neurologist is also important to monitor the child's condition and adjust treatment as needed.

Avoid attempting to restrain your youngster. Don't try to push anything into your child's mouth; instead, let the seizure run its course while you leave him on the ground. After the seizure is over, let your child sleep if he wants to. If this is your child's first seizure, take him to the doctor right away. Just make sure his airway is clear to prevent choking.

CHAPTER TEN: BATTLING ASTHMA

Does your child occasionally wheeze and feel chest pain or tightness? Does he have trouble breathing? Or perhaps he has a persistent cough. A youngster with asthma has sensitive, irritated airways. It affects roughly 20% of Singaporean youngsters, making it quite widespread.

What to Do: ⬛ Immediately follow your child's doctor's advice and have him use an inhaler. Avoid common triggers like dust, pollen, animal fur, tobacco smoke, and stress. Repetition of the procedure every 20 to 60 minutes to an hour is advised. Bring your child to the doctor right away if the asthma symptoms are not relieved or have worsened, or if they return within four hours.

Helping your child fight asthma

There are several ways to help your child with asthma manage his condition:

Create an asthma action plan with his doctor. This plan should include information on how to recognize the signs of an asthma attack, what to do in case of an attack, and how to properly use any medications.

Make sure the child takes his medications as prescribed. This includes both preventative medications and quick-relief medications.

Teach the child how to use an inhaler properly. This will help ensure that they are getting the proper amount of medication.

Help the child avoid triggers that may cause an asthma attack. Common triggers include dust, mold, pet dander, and smoking.

Help the child maintain a healthy lifestyle. This includes regular physical activity, a well-balanced diet, and getting enough rest.

Keep the child's doctor informed of any changes in their condition or symptoms. Regular check-ups and monitoring of the child's asthma can help ensure that treatment is working and that any adjustments are made as needed.

Is your youngster or newborn not going potty as frequently as he usually does? Has his bowel movement pattern changed significantly? Are his stools harder than usual? He might be constipated. The firm abdomen, pain, and irritability are other signs. Given that breast milk is easily absorbed, constipation in breastfed infants is uncommon.

There are several ways to handle constipation in children, including:

Encouraging them to drink more water and other fluids.

Adding more fiber to their diet, such as fruits, vegetables, and whole grains.

Promoting routine physical activity

Teaching them to use the bathroom regularly, such as at the same time each day.

Using a mild laxative or stool softener under the guidance of a pediatrician.

Teaching them to relax and take their time when using the bathroom to avoid withholding behavior.

It's important to note that if the constipation persists despite these interventions or if there are other symptoms such as abdominal pain, rectal bleeding, or unexplained weight loss, it's best to consult with a pediatrician for further evaluation.

Do your child's limbs, face, or trunk have a red, itchy rash? Does he frequently scratch and whine about itches? Children who have eczema typically have a family history of the disorder as well as other linked illnesses like asthma or hay fever. It's not contagious.

Eczema Cause In Children

The exact cause of eczema in children is not fully understood, but it is believed to be a combination of genetic and environmental factors. A defect in the skin barrier can cause the skin to become dry, itchy, and easily irritated. This defect can be inherited and run in families. Environmental factors such as exposure to certain irritants, allergens, or stress can also trigger eczema symptoms. Additionally, certain skin bacteria and a dysfunction of the immune system may also play a role in the development of eczema.

What to Do: ▯ Keep your child's skin moisturized and apply a topical steroid cream as directed by the doctor. ▯ Giving your child an antihistamine (anti-itch medication) before bed will help him feel less itchy and sleep better.

▯ Keep away from typical triggers such unexpected temperature changes, dust, fur, tobacco smoke, and stress.

Bring your child to the doctor if the itching interferes with his daily activities or sleep, or if there are crusting or seeping sores. ▯ Use gentle soaps; ▯ Dress your child in light cotton clothing.

CONCLUSION

As advised, asking questions about the condition and available treatments and maintaining open lines of communication with your child's healthcare professional are crucial for managing your child's condition.

Make sure your youngster is aware of the disease management strategy you've developed.

Be empathetic and supportive of your child's emotions.

Make sure you and your child are informed on the sickness and how to handle it.

Keep a positive outlook and try to keep your youngster as active and involved in their regular activities as you can.

Ensure that your child takes all recommended drugs on time, and monitor any changes in their symptoms.

Speak with other parents, your family, and organizations that can offer resources and information to get assistance.

As a parent, look after yourself so that you can be there for your child.

Having some knowledge of the sickness is also a good idea if you want to manage your child's illness.

It is advised to inform the child's doctor of any changes to their condition or symptoms. Regular examinations and monitoring of the child's condition can help ensure that the medication is effective and that any necessary corrections are made.